Mental Models

The super guide to improving decision making, problem solving and logic analysis.

Better decisions, clearer thinking, and greater self-awareness.

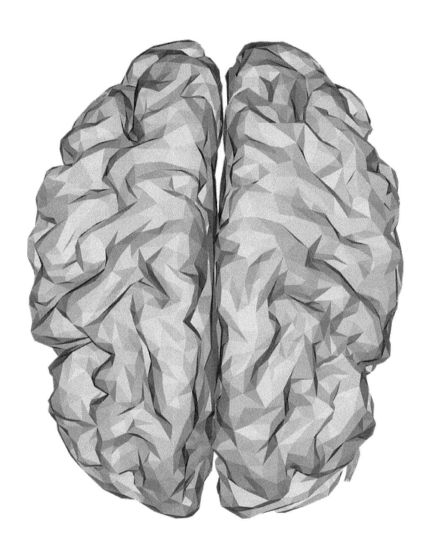

Table of Contents

INTRODUCTION 9

CHAPTER 1: INTRODUCTION TO MENTAL MODELS 11

CHAPTER 2: HOW TO HAVE CLEAR THINKING? 14

CHAPTER 3: IMPORTANCE OF CRITICAL THINKING SKILLS 19

CHAPTER 4: WHAT IS YOUR MENTAL MODEL? 34

CHAPTER 5: HOW TO BE OPEN-MINDED? 39

CHAPTER 6: SPEND THE TIME WISELY 53

CHAPTER 7: GETS BETTER DECISION MAKING 63

CHAPTER 8: HOW TO SEE MORE CLEARLY? 81

CHAPTER 9: LEARNING ORGANIZATION 90

CHAPTER 10: BECOME ONE WITH NATURE 103

© Copyright 2019 by Luis Ethan - All rights reserved.

The following Book is reproduced below with the goal of providing information that is as accurate and reliable as possible. Regardless, purchasing this Book can be seen as consent to the fact that both the publisher and the author of this book are in no way experts on the topics discussed within and that any recommendations or suggestions that are made herein are for entertainment purposes only. Professionals should be consulted as needed prior to undertaking any of the action endorsed herein.

This declaration is deemed fair and valid by both the American Bar Association and the Committee of Publishers Association and is legally binding throughout the United States.

Furthermore, the transmission, duplication, or reproduction of any of the following work including specific information will be considered an illegal act irrespective of if it is done electronically or in print. This extends to creating a secondary or tertiary copy of the work or a recorded copy and is only allowed with the express written consent from the Publisher. All additional right reserved.

The information in the following pages is broadly considered a truthful and accurate account of facts and as such, any inattention, use, or misuse of the information in question by the reader will render any resulting actions solely under their purview. There are no scenarios in which the publisher or the original author of this work can be in any fashion deemed liable for any hardship or damages that may befall them after undertaking information described herein.

Additionally, the information in the following pages is intended only for informational purposes and should thus be thought of as universal. As befitting its nature, it is presented without assurance regarding its prolonged validity or interim quality. Trademarks that are mentioned are done without written consent and can in no way be considered an endorsement from the trademark holder.

Introduction

"Two heads are better than one," many people say. It's no surprise because our own biases and experiences limit us. We also lack the areas of expertise, which results in the development and priority of mental models that you might not realize in the first place.

For example, there are two employees. The first one excels in sales while the latter remains superb in other business aspects. When both of them work together, their combined insights can crack a challenge. However, it's not always possible to host a discussion when making a crucial decision. As a professional, it's important to think about the problem yourself. But the good news is that there's an excellent way to maximize your decision-making, commonly called mental models.

You probably have heard it before. But what is a mental model? How can you navigate your mental model? Good questions. You have come to the right place! In this eBook, you will know everything about mental modes! Are you ready? Take a close look at the following.

Chapter 1: Introduction to Mental Models

Known as an explanation of how something works, a mental model is considered an overarching term for framework, concept, or worldview. Called as a representation of the surrounding world, a mental model tells about the relationship between its parts and an individual's perception of his actions and consequences.

Mental models can help everyone understand life. The supply and demand, for example, is a mental model that supports individuals to elucidate and comprehend how the economy works. Game theory is also a mental model that enables a person to understand trust and relationship.

Mental models serve as a guide to one's behavior or perception. They act as a thinking tool that a person uses to make decisions, solve daily problems, and understand life as a whole. That's why learning a new model gives everyone the chance to perceive the world differently.

Despite intensive development, mental models remain imperfect but useful. A mental model in engineering or physics, for instance, doesn't provide an error-free explanation of the universe. However, the best mental methods from such disciplines have enabled professionals and other experts to build high-end bridges, develop innovative technologies, explore the outer space, and many more. *"Scientists agree that there's no 100% correct theory,"* according to historian Yuval Noah Harari. *"The test of knowledge is about utility. It goes beyond the truth,"* he added.

The best mental models are the ideas that a person employs the most. In general, they are useful in everyday living, and a clearer understanding will help someone to take good actions and make smart decisions. That's why developing and growing a base of mental models can play a critical role in rational and effective thinking.

As with a personal algorithm, mental models can help set an approach to handling and addressing a problem. They can also shape one's behavior, enabling a person to live life to the fullest. They can even play a big role in reasoning, cognition, and decision-making. *"The mind is able to build small-scale models to anticipate and deal with new events,"* Kenneth Craik said.

Experts believed that mental models have originated with Kenneth Craik's The Nature of Explanation in 1943. Published in 1927, Georges-Henri Luquet argued that a child could build internal models and the view has relatively influenced a number of psychologists, including Jean Piaget.

In 1983, Philip Johnson-Laird also published a book about mental models. In the same year, Albert Stevens and Deidre Gentner edited different chapters in a book entitled Mental Models.

Since then, the use of the idea in several fields has been prevalent, and Donald Norman is one of the researchers. The term situation model was first used by Teun A. van Dijk and Walter Kinstsch, and wherein they showed the importance of the thinking tools for discourse production and comprehension.

Chapter 2: How to Have Clear Thinking?

Called as a reasoning unclouded by prejudices and fears, clear thinking means accepted facts or assumptions. It is considered the ability to think critically or engage reflectively. An individual who has a good memory or can accumulate information is not a clear thinker.

Clear thinking is the capacity to deduce consequences and use the information to address a problem. It helps us acquire new knowledge and make smart life decisions. Clear thinkers can understand the connections between various ideas. They can determine, create, and assess arguments. They can detect inconsistencies in reasoning, address problems systematically, ascertain the relevance of ideas, perceive the world accurately, hypothesize, and reflect on their beliefs.

Clear thinking also plays a critical role in everyone's longevity or lifestyle. The clearer our thought, the better will be our capacity to perceive, put an end to everyday challenges, and become self-aware. The skill translates into wiser decisions regarding a person's personal achievements, interpersonal relationships, and purpose. More than that, clear thinking improves our contributions in the workplace and society as a whole. It also improves lifestyle and longevity.

However, different factors affect clear thinking. A place, for instance, can extremely influence your mind.

Time is also a big factor. The food you take, the past impressions, and actions can impact a person's way of thinking. So, how to have clear thinking? Remember that the clarity of thinking is not instant. It's a long and stressful process. It does not happen overnight. As time passes by, an individual can foster his mind, increasing efficiency and productivity. To develop clear thinking, there are many helpful ways to follow. But the following list is the most acceptable and common steps to take into consideration. Read on for more information!

Check one's Attitude

It cannot be denied that focus follows an individual's desires. A person can think of new ideas and ways when he wants to achieve a goal in the first place.

On the other hand, a professional only think of reasons why it is not a perfect idea to pursue his goals when he lacks passion. To attain clear thinking, be honest about your desire. Do you want it? Do you do it because it's what you enjoy the most? Whatever the case may be, it will save your time at the beginning of all your pursuits.

Be Clear With Your Purpose

As with other goals, you have to be specific to achieve clear thinking. Sometimes, we may keep changing our objectives, which in turn can demand our brain to change its concentration and lose our path. To keep anyone's focus, sit for a minute or two, and write down. Think about what you want to achieve and stick to it. It's normal to get distracted in the midst of your journey. Just reflect on your purpose because it helps.

Take Advantage of Your Passion for managing Emotions

As you strive to turn clear thinking into a reality, your desire overcomes the challenges. However, these problems can overwhelm your emotions. This is especially true when a person suffers from a recent, potential loss.

To keep one's focus, look ahead to make your dreams a reality. Also, use your passion to control or manage your emotions.

Use Negative Thinking to Make a Smart Decision and a Positive Action

Negative thinking leads to a terrible negativity. It frees an individual's imagination to achieve what he wants in the beginning.

But negative thinking can also be an advantage. To produce a positive action, take advantage of the *'Why not = How to'* technique.

For example, you are unable to make a bright decision, solve the problem systematically, or evaluate arguments.

Many would see these weaknesses negatively. Of course, you would feel the same thing at first. But use them as a signpost to plan to reach your dreams.

To make a smart decision or handle a problem well, connect and weigh different ideas in mind. Reflect on your own values and beliefs. Detect the top mistakes in your reasoning. Plus, determine the importance of an idea. But you cannot do it on your own sometimes. Seek assistance from a colleague, friend, or family.

Use your Logic in Important Situations

Many of us can start with a clear focus. But we may be diverted by others, which in turn can affect our direction. To retain clear concentration and thinking, focus on the issue, and see the difference in every conversation. Don't just concentrate on the ego itself.

What does it mean? Or how does it work? In all conversations, make sure to concentrate on the issue you want to achieve. Don't direct your attention on your egos to reach your goal objectively.

Chapter 3: Importance of Critical Thinking Skills

As you master critical thinking skills, learn to understand logical connections between ideas, identify mistakes in reasoning, solve problems systematically or hypothesize, there's a multitude of benefits you can reap. The most common is to make a better decision. When you face a predicament about life's purpose, interpersonal relationships, or personal achievement, you can make a smart decision.

Here are the other importance of critical thinking skills:

It Develops or Encourages Curiosity

Curiosity stands beyond a profound understanding of what surrounds us. But it encourages us to go out of our comfort zone and seek other information to hone our skillset over time. A teacher, for example, looks for something new to provide effective, timely, and fun instruction.

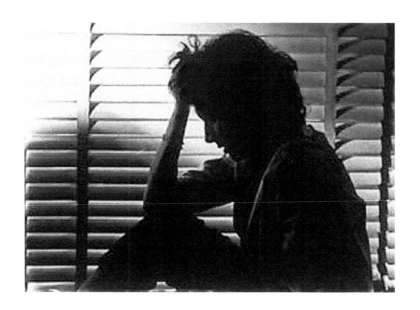

Critical thinkers remain inquisitive about a variety of topics and have wide interests. They remain curious about the world and the people. Aside from the understanding, they have an appreciation for other people's beliefs, views, or cultures, which makes them a lifelong learner. Since they are curious by nature, they apply clear thinking skills every moment. They are alert for an opportunity to apply their thinking habits in different situations. The desire to think of the simplest issues clearly can show their interests to receive constructive results.

Critical or clear thinkers always ask the following questions:

- Why is it necessary? Who is the affected part of the community?
- Is there something I overlook? What's hidden?
- Why should I listen to this professional? What learning can I acquire?
- What else should I take into consideration?

Critical thinkers don't stop asking questions. They enjoy exploring each side of a specific issue instead. They also love to elucidate deeper facts in all available data.

It Fosters Creativity or Imagination

Below problem solving, creativity is the second top skill that every child should learn, according to educators. It's no surprise because effective critical thinkers are largely creative individuals and creativity has defined itself as an essential skill in the modern workforce.

Clear thinking in marketing and business relies on a person's ability to be creative. When companies get the most out of their creativity throughout product development, they can stand out from the competition and succeed in the marketplace.

Creative people also question assumptions about different things. Rather than arguing for limitations, they ask *"why not"* or *"how?"* called eternal, which indicates that every individual is unlimited. What's surprising is that they don't get stuck in their comfort zone. They go out that comforting cocoon to learn new things, develop skills, unleash new capabilities, and become a versatile professional over time.

It Develops and Strengthens Problem-Solving Ability

Do you know that critical thinker are likely to be problem-solvers? Yes, it's a fact, and it's the most important skill that every learner should have in order to face future challenges and come up with imaginative solutions.

Albert Einstein, one of the most prolific investors, said that he's not so smart: it's just that he stayed with a problem longer. When given an hour to address a problem, he'd spend 5 minutes on the solution and the rest for research purposes. This kind of commitment and patience indicates the quality of what an effective critical thinker is. This is the reason why a critical thinking ability can play a big role in becoming a good problem solver.

Developing a clear and critical thinking ability prepares everyone to face complex predicaments in the coming years. Whether it's global warming, overpopulation, pollution, energy crises, electronic waste management or water shortages, critical thinkers can produce lasting and innovative solutions to alleviate or put an end to these never-ending issues.

It's Considered a Multi-Faceted Practice

Known for encompassing a range of disciplines, critical thinking can cultivate a wide array of cognitive talents. It's indeed a cross-curricular activity for the mind, which must be exercised to function at its best.

Critical thinking promotes the development of other skills. These can include analytical thinking, reasoning skills, evaluative skills, planning skills, logical thinking, open-mindedness, observational skills, self-reflective capacity, language skills, decision making, questioning ability, creative visualization strategies, and more.

It Develops Independence

One of the primary goals of education is to train young students to think independently. When they start to think for themselves, they become independent, responsible, and ready to adjust in the modern and fast-paced industry.

Independent thinking skills are usually at the forefront of learning how to be a great thinker and effective leader. Independent thinkers learn how to make sense of what surrounds them based on observation and personal experience. In most cases, they can make critical and well-informed decisions, gain confidence, and learn from mistakes.

When individuals think critically, they do it in a self-directed manner. While the style of thinking is disciplined, it becomes a great self-correcting mindset. As they continue to develop the skills thru experience, the abilities can become second nature.

As stated earlier, independent thinking skills are among the competencies all educators strive to inculcate in every young student's mind. They do that to provide learners a gift they can use for a lifetime. Once they graduate, they can pursue their dreams with pride and confidence.

It's a Lifelong Skill

Lower order thinking skills prepare a student for today. Critical thinking and other higher-order competencies, on the contrary, prepare everyone for long-term success as they can adjust in a different setting outside the walls of the classroom. They can handle a range of situations in the workplace, finish their job well, become productive, and acquire a lucrative career. Although it is a long process to achieve these thinking abilities, the efforts are worth it.

It Plays a Vital Role in the New Knowledge-Economy

The new knowledge economy is driven by IT. Every professional need to deal with the everyday changes, and the economy places high demands on the competency to analyze information and incorporate sources of knowledge to solve problems. Superb critical thinking promotes such skills, which can come into play in this fast-paced workplace.

It Enhances Language Skills

Clear thinking can improve the way you express your ideas. Every time you face a group of people for a presentation, you will be as eloquent and accurate as possible. In analyzing the logical structure of texts and other relevant pieces of information, critical thinking can boost comprehension abilities, which can save your time and maximize results.

It is Crucial for Self-Reflection

To structure a meaningful life according to your desires, justifying and reflecting on your values, decisions, and beliefs can make a huge difference. To do that, critical thinking serves as a perfect tool for self-evaluation, especially during a failure or even success. Do you miss something important? What would you do to realize your goals? Ask these questions when you self-reflect.

It Enhances Academic Performance

"Students who know how to critique or analyze ideas can make connections across several disciplines. They can see knowledge as applicable to everyday living and understand any type of content on a longer-lasting and more profound level," Richard Paul and Linda Elder, Authors of Critical Thinking Development: A Stage Theory said. This ability could help people of all ages to understand or fix a problem, which in turn can ensure a great academic performance or productivity. Without enough critical thinking skills, a person would find it hard to analyze his surrounding world, which can result in slow performance.

It Increases Awareness Between a Rational Thought and an Emotional Response

Knowing the difference between an emotional response and a rational thought is difficult. A critical thinker, on the other hand, makes it easy and simple. Through personal bias and careful consideration, they know how the former differs from the latter.

Emotion is considered the foe of reason. By understanding your perspective, you can consider other's point of view. Then, you can make a conclusion according to facts, not feelings.

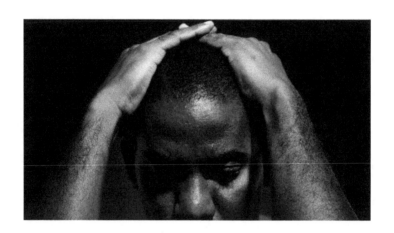

It Guarantees a Great Hiring Opportunity

Nowadays, the number of employers who look for professionals with good thinking skills has been skyrocketing. It's no wonder because they can learn quickly, solve daily problems, analyze information, and think creatively. Although those with specialized academic skills sound in-demand, a critical thinker always has the edge over the other applicants.

It can be a Deciding Factor for a Promotion

Most high-paying jobs, these days, require higher-order thinking skills, which can include generating effective ideas and making smart decisions. More often than not, job interviewers ask applicants with questions that examine and test their ability. When seeking a promotion, these competencies will be of great help.

It Makes One's Approach

With critical thinking skills, critical thinkers are aware of different approaches on how to solve a problem. They can evaluate each approach critically. Instead of depending on a standard problem-solving method. They identify other valuable and effective techniques to increase productivity and success.

It Saves Time

As a critical thinker, you're certain that not all information is relevant to your problem-solving and decision making. However, some don't know how to get rid of any irrelevant data. Critical thinking skills teach you how to prioritize both of your resources and time. Then, you can analyze and assess what is important to the process, which helps you know whether or not a decision is a good one.

It Leads to Autonomous Learning

Instead of relying on teachers, students with a high level of critical thinking become self-directed and independent learners. Critical thinking skills allow students to evaluate their learning styles, weaknesses, and strength. These also enable them to take ownership or be responsible for their education. Students in an English class, for example, might write a reflective essay about how their writing skills have improved and what they need to focus on. This allows them to view their performance and reach good conclusions.

From solving problems in school to facing real-life situations, critical thinking skills enable the youth and professionals to present their ideas well. Instead of accepting their personal reasoning, they make a research, look for statistics, and other important data to prove their stance. Clear thinking can also result in empathy for other people's point of view and better control of one's learning.

It Brings New Ideas

When a potential issue exists in the workplace, many would assume that it falls under a predetermined category. Some who possess superb critical thinking don't make assumptions. Using their logical skills, they remove the temptation to classify a problem under a common problem in the past. Then, it forces managers and employees to look beyond traditional solutions and new ideas to address a predicament and achieve meaningful results.

It Promotes Other Options

Another advantage of critical thinking is that it enables a company to develop a variety of realistic and feasible solutions to address an issue. This allows businesses of all sizes to provide various solutions to prospective clients, and it also leads to effective innovation. With different solutions to a specific problem, a company can address a dilemma with the use of existing resources, saving their time, effort, and cash as well.

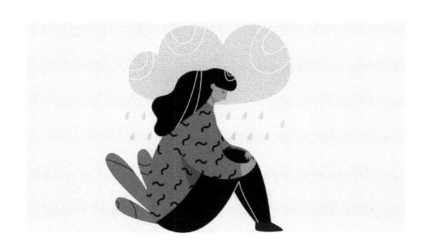

Chapter 4: What is Your Mental Model?

There are many mental models that people use every day, in which they don't realize in the first place. When we interpret the world or understand the relationship between things, our mental models come into play. When we face new life experiences or a problem, these thinking tools can make a critical role.

As we're born, we already have a mental model. As the years pass by, it becomes effectively strong and stable. Then, our mind unleashes or designs another mental model. As we learn and acquire experiences, our base of mental models becomes broader, which in turn can enable us to think clearly and rationally.

The world is, no doubt a complicated place, and trying to understand it leads to confusion. More than that, individuals learn to accept their limitations. While these can be a disadvantage, they provide professionals with opportunities to strengthen their weaknesses, foster strengths, become a critical thinker, and turn a high level of performance into a reality.

You probably are wondering what your mental models are. While some are considered common knowledge, others are sophisticated, and the latticework they produce is intimidating to deal with. Don't worry! You're not alone! Most beginners and even seasoned critical thinkers experience the same thing.

The most common mental model is Murphy's Law. Known as an optimistic law, the metal model states that if anything can go wrong, it surely will. Murphy's Law also indicates that if there are two ways to do something, and one of them can lead to a big mess, a person will still do it. But its explosive nature is the idea that someone will make the wrong choice whatever his decisions to take.

Occam razor is another mental model to know. Although it's difficult as it sounds, it states that the simplest explanation is the correct one. When a person tries to understand what really happened, the development of the most basic hypothesis can help.

Hanlon's razor is another common mental model that we might have. What does it mean? And how does it work? A marketing qualified lead, for example, goes dark at some point during the acquisition process. Then, you might assume that the client doesn't want to continue. However, Hanlon's Razor asks everyone not to attribute to malice what could be explained by carelessness. Instead, it's realistic to assume that the person has a hectic schedule.

Pareto principle, on the other hand, is commonly called as the 80/20 rule, which means the results are not properly distributed. For instance, 20% of your time produces approximately 80% of the results and 20% of the work leads to 89% of the returns. If you can hone on the necessary skills, the success rate is higher than you have ever thought. But it's easier said than done. It is a long and stressful process, which requires one's patience, commitment, and persistence.

Another mental model is Sturgeon's law, which means 90% of everything is considered crap. That's why you have to be selective with both of your energy and time. How to begin? Start with the non-crap and then find your way out. While some are likely to rush, get the process done as slowly as possible. Unlike the Pareto Principle, it is a more restrictive version in most cases.

Last but not least is Parkinson Law. Compared to other mental models, it is quite different, which indicates that triviality can set in easily because it feels great to voice a person's opinion and feel productive. When your mental model is similar to Parkinson law, reflect on your top priorities. Then, ask if your actions are relevant to your goals. From there, work expands to fill your time and remember that working at a relaxed pace can result in self-sabotage.

To know more information about the common and popular mental models, read on! We discussed other thinking tools in detail in the succeeding chapters.

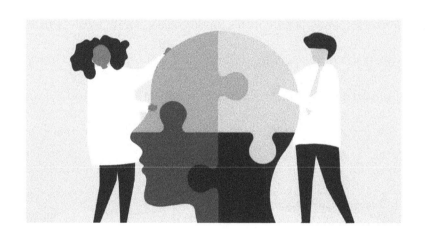

Chapter 5: How to be Open-Minded?

While mental models refer to the representation of the surrounding world, open-mindedness is about the ability of a person to adopt assumptions based on a changing circumstance at work or in other places. Since the working environment leads to new occurrences, individuals are unable to reach expectations and make the objectives happen.

The application of open-mindedness, however, makes the mind flexible to overcome a specific situation, which in turn can bring academic performance and productivity up to the highest level. How's it possible? Well, by changing the assumptions and adopting relevant suppositions, it could be a reality.

Unlike mental models, open-mindedness leads to the flexibility of the mind to adopt assumptions, which can enable them to solve existing challenges in their daily living. Because of the complexity of the 21st business environment, companies look for critical thinking and open-minded professional.

But how to be open-minded? As with mental models, acquiring quality takes time and attention; it also requires a lifelong process for someone to develop the in-demand skill in the workplace, studies, and another environment.

To be open-minded, everyone might find it tough because most of us set a certain comfort in our mind that's hard to break. However, opening the mind to new opportunities, adventure, relationships, and knowledge can bring a greater sense of happiness or fulfillment to your daily living. Before anything else, find your motivation. For everyone to make it possible to embrace and accept new ideas, it's imperative to motivate oneself to try different things. Ask why do you want to become open-minded? Are you committed to accepting different assumptions from your colleagues and other people that surround you? Are you more than willing to take action to turn this goal into a reality? Then, you probably are ready.

After that, it's a perfect time to choose specific areas to develop. Which life areas do you want to open up to ideas? For example, if you're eating the same food all the time, you perhaps like to try some variation. You can give at least one recipe or food a shot every week. It's a realistic and simple approach, after all.

While many would aim high, don't do the same thing. Start from a small goal because you might not be ready to experience a sudden and big change in your life. That's why chunk your objectives into small pieces to make this approach reliable and realistic.

After finding your motivation and choosing the areas to develop, your job does not stop there. In fact, it's just the beginning of your journey towards becoming an open-minded individual. Before we learn how to become open-minded, below are some benefits of having an open mind:

Let Go of Control

Close-minded people don't grow personally and professionally. They believe they are higher than anyone else in terms of expertise, knowledge, and experience. But the truth is that they don't grow as a professional. Open-minded, on the other hand, individuals have the opportunity to be in control of their thoughts. They allow themselves to acquire new ideas and challenge their existing beliefs.

"Nothing permanent in this world but change," everyone says. Every second, the workplace, the school, and other places change. So, close-minded individuals are unable to adapt to new trends, making their knowledge obsolete. But the ability to accept assumptions, facts, or opinions enable them to be flexible and effective.

Experience Change

Opening up your mind to new thoughts gives you the chance to change how you perceive the world. But this doesn't mean it will change your existing beliefs and perspectives. Sometimes, the process may just strengthen your mental faculties, and open-mindedness allows you to achieve stronger outcomes and a fulfilling life.

More often than not, some are afraid to adapt the latest trends or innovation. It's no surprise because they are not ready to fail. They think that accepting other's ideas and failing make them incapable or ineffective. But we're not perfect after all. Some are good in math, while others are poor. Although you struggle with numbers, you may be good in other fields. So, consider the latest change or ideas as an opportunity to foster and become more competitive in the coming years. Take them seriously and find your own ways for personal and professional development.

When someone suggests an idea, don't feel negative about it. In fact, you can consider yourself lucky because a thought from peers and superiors can help you bridge the gap, identify a better solution, save your time, and maximize a perfect result at the end of the day.

Make Yourself Vulnerable

It's scary to discern the world thru an open mind because you show your vulnerability to others. You also admit that you lack in terms of knowledge and performance. The process can be exhilarating and confusing, as well.

But it's good to know that making yourself vulnerable can be a good thing. First, you will learn different things, develop your skills, meet expectations, and bring your knowledge up to the highest level. Second, the process becomes easier than expected while you get as competitive as possible. Last but not least is that your relationship with your colleagues, peers, and other people that surround you will be meaningful. So, don't be skeptical to look vulnerable. With the help of others and your persistence to excellence, your weaknesses will surely be your strengths in the future. But don't heavily rely on colleagues. Remember that learning by doing is better, which in turn can lead to productivity, effectiveness, and flexibility.

Make Mistakes

Committing mistakes is embarrassing but a great learning experience. However, many professionals, business owners, or students don't grow after a failure and end up staying in their comfort zone. If you experience the same thing, you're not alone. Instead of lingering on a failure, consider it a learning experience for you to be a better version of yourself. What you need to do after a failure is to reflect. Did you overlook something important? What resources did you miss? From there, you'd realize why you make a mistake. Also, other people are more than willing to provide a constructive criticism. Although it hurts and affects your self-confidence, don't feel down because it's part of the process. As long as you exert effort to improve your weaknesses, you can handle the same problem easily and effectively.

Strengthen your Weaknesses

You probably are expert in communication skills, presentation, or language. Perhaps, you're poor in critical thinking activities. To strengthen yourself, being open-minded provides you a platform to acquire and build upon a base of ideas from reliable professionals. As years pass by, every thought you collect from others adds up. This strengthens your skills, enables you to acquire a new ability, and improves your limitations.

But remember that building on experiences is hard without an open mind. When you receive a feedback from superiors, take it as a constructive criticism. It hurts but looks at it positively. Also, it's essential to read in the library or online. For those who don't have ample time to go to the nearest library, turn on your phone and browse the internet with a click of a button.

Gain Confidence

Close-minded individuals are confined by their own beliefs or other's perspectives. Open-mindedness, on the contrary, enables you to have a strong sense of yourself. This means you can boost the level of your self-esteem. When you're in front of a big crowd, you can carry yourself well. For a presentation and other activities, you can perform according to your goals and other standards.

Close-minded people lack confidence. In fact, they stay in their comfort zone and believe that their knowledge is unmatched. But the truth is that most of their skills need improvement. For you to boost your self-esteem, start to be open-minded, and don't stop learning.

Be Honest As much As Possible

Close-minded people are not honest enough to admit that they lack the skills. Individuals with an open mind are different. At first, they admit that the level of their knowledge is far from perfection, and this understanding leads to a sense of authenticity. When you're honest with your capabilities, many would love to give you a hand, which can establish a good rapport in the long run. Whenever you go, you can build a fun relationship with others, establishing a fun and competitive working environment.

For some, being open-minded is as easy as eating a pie. For others, it's a real headache. It's something they need to think constantly and make an effort to obtain. However, thinking openly and embracing new ideas will produce benefits for both of your career and life.

Since you struggle to face the challenge, what are you going to do next? Here are what you can use or adapt to be open-minded in 2019 and beyond. Are you ready? Take a close look at the following:

Talk Less and Listen More

Before you can covey your real message, you have to seek first to understand. We don't specifically learn new things when we talk more. By listening intently and silently, we can acquire fresh ideas. When interacting with other people, listen profoundly for at least 70% of your time. Don't use your phone or stop multitasking. That way, you can focus and learn new ideas and approaches, which are a key for personal and professional development.

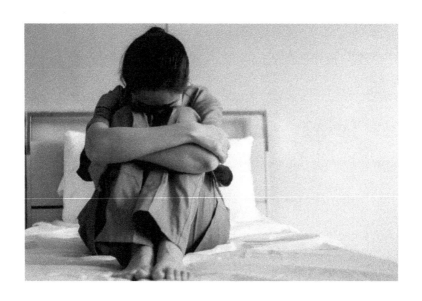

Avoid Snap Decisions

How many times has an event hit you straight directly in your blood pressure? Does the email go unreturned? Does a call go unanswered? Do you learn a bad surprise thru a memo or second party? Whatever the case may be, most of us react to an unexpected as immediately as possible. But is it a good idea? Well, making snap decisions is not a smart action. Instead of showing anger or judgment, get the facts first. Don't be deceived by your emotions. Control and gather everything you need. This can guarantee a good flow, promote a stress-free environment, and boost productivity.

Show your Earnest Gratitude to People's Suggestions

There are several causes of consternation in any settings. The lack of gratitude for an idea is among them. It's normal to feel a sense of injustice when colleagues steal a specific employee's ideas. But will they be likely to offer their critical thinking again? Of course, not. They will save their ideas for another company where they feel appreciated and respected for their job. As a colleague and professional, bear this courtesy in mind.

Encourage Frankness and Don't Be Afraid to Handle It

Have you ever received a straight and straightforward feedback? What did you feel? Did you feel hurt? Or were you unwillingly accepted what you have heard? Then, remember that sensitive feelings can relatively influence your performance in school, at home, or in the workplace. To reduce the impact, accept it. Then, start to take a criticism constructively. When you meet someone who couldn't accept the truth regarding his performance, be wary when giving your feedback. Make sure to incorporate high tact and diplomacy. Respect for the person should be noticeable and obvious. If you master this ability, your skill to speak, hear, and share with an open mind will make the impossible possible.

Look for Other Opportunities

One of the results of being open-minded is the ability to seek or discover opportunities and approaches to addressing everyday challenges.

It's normal to think that there are no available ideas. But look at every possibility and angle to put an end to a problem.

Thomas Edison has earned worldwide popularity because of its lightbulb. But he had attempted a thousand times before he perfected his invention according to reports and studies.

Another inventor who had the same trait is Colonel Sanders, in which he tried his chicken recipe for approximately 1,009 times according to sources. When you learn to accept new opportunities, you will never get tired to make an effort to fulfill your dreams. If you feel hopeless, don't rush. Pause, think, and start again.

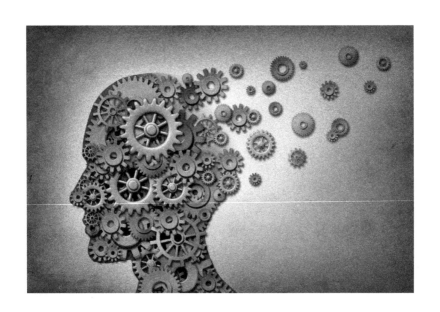

Chapter 6: Spend the Time Wisely

A good time management leads to more productivity. Professionals at home or in the office are able to get more things done compared to those who can't spend their time wisely. They have more energy for everything they need to fulfil. They feel less stressed and relate positively to everyone around them. They also feel better about themselves, enabling them to live life to the fullest and experience a deep sense of fulfillment. However, managing or spending your time wisely is easier said than done. In fact, it depends on skills learned thru planning, self-control, evaluation, and self-analysis. Some strategies work best for you. But it depends on your level of discipline, personality, and ability to motivate yourself.

The mental model can also come into play. But what kind of mental model that can enable you to manage your time? This is where the Pareto Principle has got anyone's back. In chapter 4, we have learned that the mental model is known as the 80/20 rule. Used to analyze tasks or manage workload, the Pareto Principle is one of the most useful techniques for spending time properly.

But how the 80/20 rule gives clarity to a person's life? Generally speaking, you can incorporate the principle into your personal life to alleviate inefficiency and maximize productivity. How are you going to do it? Let's get started!

- These days, let's accept the fact that we spend a lot of time using our phone. We always open one or more apps for entertainment and information. Well, it's a bad idea. Figure out the apps you use most of the time. Then, delete what's unnecessary. From there, you would see a big difference in the time you save and use for productive activities.

- In the workplace, imagine you are bombarded with different tasks every day. How are you going to deal with it? At first, it's overwhelming and tiring. But identify 20% of the tasks that are extremely important and make sure it brings 80% of the results. Having said that, you can manage or prioritize your daily activities in the office better. This helps you get the most of your time, reduces effort, and leads to good outcomes.

- Most of us like to wear the same clothes on a regular basis. It's about time to give your wardrobe a rest. Start from decluttering your closet by donating some of your unused dresses to charity to free up your mind as well.

- There's probably a number of video games and television shows that account for the 80% of your time. So, pick your top favorites and stop jumping from a game to another.

- It's estimated that approximately 80% of your money is spent on unnecessary things. Sometimes, you go to the mall without a list of stuff to buy. Also, other people get tempted to try things they are neither useful nor imperative. The secret here is to make a list, stick to it, and create a careful budget planning.

Applying the 80/20 Rule for Effective Time Management

Whether you're aiming to manage your time or set a goal, you can enjoy many benefits when you apply the mental model effectively. While some make big and drastic changes, don't do the same thing because it's unrealistic and impossible to achieve. Little changes in your habits or lifestyle are a good start. If you are quite confused about how to apply the 80/20 rule, don't worry as here are some easy and quick tips to bear in mind:

Start and Finish the Hardest Tasks

There are different kinds of employees in the workforce. Some seem super-busy and work day and night without finishing every assigned and urgent task. Others finish everything ahead of time and look for other duties to handle.

Which of these best represents you as an employee? If you relate yourself to the former, don't lose hope or feel stressed with your situation. First, understand that the case happens when you do low-priority tasks. Look for something that will add real value to your work instead. Then, start with a complex task. Although it might consume most of your time, all your efforts will pay off at the end of the day. While it's tempting to do small and simple things, make the hardest activities a top priority.

Stick to Your Main Goal

What makes successful people different from others? Attitude comes first. When setting goals, they work on it despite the failures. When it comes to their time, they are likely to be intentional on how it is utilized. Even though it is tempting to indulge in gossips, side-talks, or distractions, they are focused. Then, they never lose track of their development and progress. Of course, everyone wants to be successful and wealthy. So, what's the secret? Keep your eyes on your goal, use Pareto's principle, and don't lose hope despite the failures. Take them positively and exert more effort to manage your time and make your dreams happen.

Determine what Affects your Concentration

Staying focused on your task is hard, especially when there are distractions around you. You're not alone because most employees and even students find distractions the main roadblock to productivity. But some colleagues have their way out with distractions. So, if they can, you can do the same thing.

Of course, every item has a deadline, so getting distracted is something you cannot afford. To keep your focus, keep your phone on a silent mode to avoid the notification sounds and make your concentration stronger. Also, we are likely to get distracted by many things. The secret here is to determine what distracts you the most. Then, try your best to keep them away. At first, it's hard. But your efforts, time, and attention will all be worth it in the future.

Other Strategies for Better Time Management

Know-How You Spend your Time

It may sound unnecessary to determine how you spend your time every day. But it's relatively helpful. To do that, simply keep a log and record what you do for 15-minute intervals for a single week or two. Then, evaluate the outcomes. To assess the results, ascertain which tasks require most of your time and identify when you are most effective. Is it your job, recreation, family, or personal?

Identifying the most time-consuming activities can enable you to identify and create a customized action. In addition, that knowledge can assist you to be realistic and specific in planning. You can also estimate ample time for other important activities.

Be Sure to Set Priorities

Spending time wisely requires a distinction between what is urgent and what is important. Professionals agree that the most important paperwork is not the most urgent task to finish. But we are likely to let the urgent dominate our everyday routine at home or in the workplace. While urgent and important tasks must be done, experts recommend that we should minimize our attention to projects that are not important despite their urgency. This allows you to keep your focus and achieve the results you desire. In addition, it enables you to control your time, maximize success, and reduce stress.

The simplest ways to prioritize is to create and develop a "to do" list. Whether you make a daily or weekly list, consider your lifestyle and rank all items in an order.

Take Advantage of a Planning Tool

Have you ever heard about personal planning tools? You can use them to boost your productivity. Good examples include pocket diaries, computer programs, calendars, index cards, electronic planners, and notebooks. Writing your tasks and schedules down can free your mind to concentrate on top of your priorities. If you are an auditory learner, you may find dictating your thoughts comfortable. To find the perfect tool, use the one that works for your situation.

Get Fully Organized

Disorganization leads to poor time management. That's why professional organizers suggest everyone remove the clutter. With unnecessary items, you may find decluttering complicated. You can set up three boxes labeled "Toss," "Keep," and "Give Away."

Discard items in the "Toss" box and include stuff in the "Give Away" box you'd like to sell. Plus, put the items you want to use in the "Keep" box. After decluttering, your job does not stop there. When the mess is gone, implement a system that enables you to handle less information.

Stop Procrastinating

Have you ever experienced putting off tasks because they seem overwhelming and confusing? You can break them down into smaller and feasible segments. When you're having a trouble on how to get started, collect materials, and organize notes. After that, build your own reward system whenever you complete a specific task.

Don't Attempt to Multi-Task

Multi-tasking can be an advantage but a problem as well. Every time you switch from one paperwork to another, you could lose your time, which can cause a loss of productivity. Recent studies show that multi-tasking does not save time. More than that, it can cause difficulties in keeping and maintaining your concentration.

Most importantly, the key to time management is discipline, commitment, patience, and persistence. Without all these qualities, you will always end up procrastinating and losing your focus.

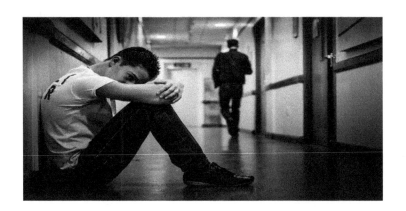

Chapter 7: Gets Better Decision Making

The ability to make a good and quick decision is essential in different life situations. To be an effective employee or professional, decision-making skills can play a critical role. Whether you love a guessing game or don't believe in your instinct, you will lose the respect of the people that surround you. More than that, your decision may ruin your expected outcome.

An excellent decision making, on the contrary, can save you time. You know which decisions to make and the ones that require further research or careful planning. You can avoid overthinking, which can save you time. The skill can also foster respect. A well-informed and confident manager in a company, for example, can earn the trust of his employees as easily as possible.

A high level of decision-making skills can serve as motivation. A person who's superb in making decisions can serve as an inspiration to others to perform and achieve. In the workplace, not all of the days are a good one. Sometimes, there are moments where your colleagues struggle to do their job, and someone else who is good in decision making can change the atmosphere.

In addition, the capacity to decide on an important issue can also prevent a potential conflict and increase productivity. While a team works in a stress-free environment, they can become as competitive as possible.

However, getting a better decision making is not as simple as everyone thinks. In fact, it takes a long but fun process. However, as with effective time management, mental models can help an individual make an ideal option despite the level of difficulty. Occam's razor is among the mental models that can play a crucial role in acquiring and mastering decision-making skills. In the previous chapter, we have also learned that Occam's Razor shows that the simplest solutions are likely to be right. Or in a different case, a person makes a choice according to the least number of assumptions, and many find it useful when they don't have the data for a well-informed decision. In such situations, most of us take the path with minimum assumptions, which introduce an error. For those who design or develop a user flow for a product, the mental model comes in handy.

Compounding is another mental model that can make a difference in one's decision making. But how does it help in better decisions? It simply allows us to realize that if we continually make good habits, those will double in the long run and support us to reach our goals within a short period.

Oftentimes, we may forget that small efforts can lead to something monumental and compounding keep our focus. No matter how difficult our goal to fulfil, we would think of the best solution to realize our dreams.

Aside from mental models, there are other ways to get better decision making. The following is a short list of steps to incorporate into your existing approaches:

Make Decision Reversible

What're the best decisions? Many would think that collecting enough information can make good career choices. Well, it can be true. However, it may affect our progress. It can even pose a danger to our lives as well.

Most successful people adopt simple and flexible heuristics to get rid of the need for deliberation in specific situations. Jeff Bezos, the founder of Amazon, asks whether a decision is reversible or irreversible, making it one of the common and popular heuristics.

What is a reversible decision? Well, it happens when someone makes it fast despite the insufficiency of information. How about an irreversible decision? It indicates that an individual slows down the process. Not only do they understand the problem, but they also ensure to consider enough evidence on their hands.

Jeff Bezos took advantage of this heuristic to found the largest online shopping platform across the world. At first, he recognized that if his pursuit of success failed, he could be able to return to his job. His decision could be considered reversible, which served him well throughout the years. In fact, the heuristic continues to pay off when Bezos makes a decision.

Decisions amidst Uncertainty

Imagine you try to eat in a new restaurant after reading an online review. Although you haven't been there, are unaware of the food, or the atmosphere is stressful, you use the information to make a decision. You even recognize that it won't be a big deal when the restaurant doesn't meet your standards.

However, uncertainty is riskier in other situations. You might take a specific job without the knowledge of the company culture.

Reversible decisions are made as quickly as possible without gathering enough information. If your decision doesn't work out, you can extract wisdom from your experience with little cost. Oftentimes, gathering information, and looking for answers are not worth the time and attention. Even though extensive research and careful planning can make your decision better, the risk of missing a chance is higher than expected.

Reverse decisions should not be an excuse to be ill-informed or act recklessly. However, it is a belief that you should adapt. Unlike irreversible decisions, reversible ones are far different. You don't need to make it like the latter.

The skill to make fast decisions can give a person a great advantage. One benefit is that small-sized businesses can move with velocity while seasoned companies move with speed. What's the difference? It indicates the difference between a failure and success.

Let's say you are headed from New York to Las Vegas and just circle around NYC for hours. It shows that you're moving with speed. However, you're not getting to your desired destination. So, speed doesn't care whether you are reaching your objectives or not.

On the contrary, velocity is different. While speed doesn't give attention to the realization of your goals, velocity requires you to move toward your dreams. That's why startups and other small businesses make quick decisions to stand apart from the competition. You can also maximize the advantage with the pace of change and other factors. The quicker you react or respond, the better the benefit you can reap.

Every decision provides us with ample data to make better choices in the future. The faster we can cycle thru the OODA loop, the better the result. While many believe that the framework is only applicable to specific situations, it is a heuristic that can play an essential part in the decision-making the process.

With enough practice and careful planning, we can become expert in identifying bad decisions, including pivoting. Aside from avoiding to stick with past choices, we can stop viewing a failure as disastrous. Then, we can view them as information that will help us make good options in the future.

Jeff Bezos compares every reversible decision to doors, which open both ways. Irreversible decisions, on the other hand, are doors that enable passage in a single direction that can get you stuck if you walk thru.

Most decisions are the reversible ones, although we can't recover both the resources and time. Plus, the reversible door provides us enough information, making us aware of what's on the different side.

Malcolm Gladwell also explains why decision making in uncertainty can be effective in his book entitled *Blink: The Power of Thinking without Thinking*. Most of us assume that sufficient information results in a better life choice. A physician, for example, suggests extra tests. Of course, we are likely to believe that additional examinations can lead to a good outcome. However, Gladwell opposes the idea. *"Everyone has to know less information to determine the signature of a phenomenon. What we need is evidence of the blood pressure, an unstable angina, fluid in the lungs, or ECG,"* he said.

"In many areas of medicine, more information does not necessarily improve the outcomes. As an example, Gladwell cites a man who arrives at a hospital with chest pains. While his vital signs don't indicate any risk factors, his lifestyle is a different case. Two years earlier, he had a serious heart operation. When the attending physician considers all available data, it seems that the person should be admitted to the hospital. Plus, the other factors are not necessary in the short term run, but he is probably at a high risk of having a cardiovascular disease over time," Gladwell added.

When you're on the lookout for a heuristic for the development of your decision making, Bezos' approach is a good strategy to use in your career and life situations. What makes his heuristic different from others is that it fights the stasis in small-sized companies and even large organizations. What matters the most is that it's effective. Although it doesn't adhere to the norm of a slow decision, Bezos' technique proves that everything is possible in making a reversible choice.

Seek Satisfaction

Another way to get better decisions is to seek satisfaction. Mostly, we get satisfied with our decisions by the process or the decision itself. Is it of high quality? Does it lead to the attainment of your goals? Does it help you get nearer in your dreams? Whatever the case may be, satisfaction in your life choices can result in a better decision making in the future.

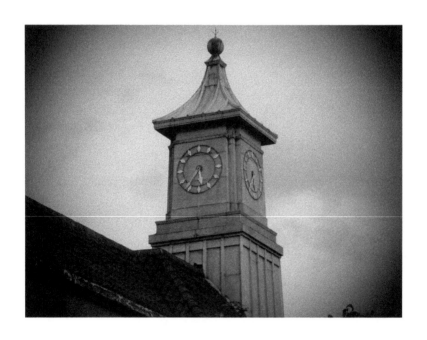

Emotions trigger how a person feels and behaves. When you're satisfied and happy with the past decisions, you can handle the same situation with a perfect choice. What will happen when you're sad and not content with your recent performance? Well, you might be willing to settle for things that don't reach your favor in the first place. When everything seems chaotic, various questions will come to your mind. Why did you make such a hasty and unplanned decision? What did you do wrong and overlook? But think again. Everything is done, and you could not travel back in time.

More than the nature of a decision, emotions can relatively affect the speed at which you make a choice. Anger can cause a rash and poor decision-making. The deep level of excitement is no exception. When you're excited, you could make decisions without weighing the implications in mind. If you feel afraid, your life choices may be filled with uncertainty, which in turn can take you longer to pick.

In addition to logic, emotion can play a critical role in helping us make good choices. Whether we understand our emotions and notice how they impact our thinking, we can manage our response and practice better options. Also, raise your logic while decreasing the emotional reactivity. You can list the pros and cons of every complicated decision because seeing every fact on a sheet of paper can aid you to think rationally about your choices. Furthermore, you can prevent emotions from enabling you to find a better version of yourself.

Don't feel Afraid and Negative on the Consequences

A person's decision entails predicting the future. In most cases, we visualize how the results of our options will make us feel and plump for the decision that can make us happy at the end of the day.

While this effective forecasting is fine, most of us can't get the most out of it. Most particularly, we tend to overestimate the effect of life events and the results of our decision. We always think that winning the lottery will make us more contented than it will in reality. *"The consequences of such events are less intense and shorter than we think,"* Daniel Gilbert, a psychologist from Harvard University, said.

What factor that leads us to come up with bad predictions? Well, the loss of aversion is the major factor. What does it mean? It's the belief that a failure will hurt more than the learning itself. Many individuals are unwilling to do a 50:50 bet except when the price is twice the amount they might lose according to Daniel Kahneman, a psychologist from Princeton University. Gilbert, together with his colleagues, shows that when people lose, they found it less painful than they have expected.

Then, Gilbert puts it down to a person's ability to rationalize every situation. *"Everyone can find new ways to see and make the world a much better place to dwell in,"* he also added.

So, what does a poor affective forecaster mean? Instead of imagining how a result might be stressful at the end of the day, look for a friend, colleague, and other peers who made the same life choice and know how they felt. Also, bear in mind that whatever your future is, it may please or hurt you. But don't play it safe. Although the failure is less risky than you think, it won't allow you to grow. It's best to commit mistakes because it becomes a great learning experience for people of all ages. Plus, don't be afraid of the consequences. Take them lightly, learn from your blunders, and become a much better professional.

Find out What Your Heart Desires

Success comes from determining your desired result. For you to fulfill your goal, you need holistic concentration. Despite the challenges along the way, don't lose sight of your specific targets.

When making choices, ask whether it is getting you closer to your objectives or it is getting you far away from your dreams. When it doesn't help you at all to make your goals happen, discard it as soon as possible. In addition, work on both of your mindset and beliefs to approach your target more effectively. While others may have failed on the same path because of weak thoughts, don't be swayed by the limitations others throw on you. Remember that a weak mind leads to poor results. Also, don't forget that attitude or winning is an option.

Establish an Effective Filter System

Does your decision only benefit yourself? Does it positively impact your family? Does it help your growth plans? Does it give other people an advantage? Whether a life choice or decision meets all these factors, you can make the perfect action, although the process is less attractive or longer.

When you don't use a filter, incorporate one approach to make good choices. After that, stick to them, whatever happens. When everything doesn't exceed your expectations, it's perhaps not ideal action.

Develop Wisdom

Every right decision always brings a good job, profound satisfaction, a lucrative career, and other rewards. How about bad life choices? Well, it still has a reward to reap. The experience itself is a good learning opportunity.

However, you can transform your daily experiences into wisdom. Just dig into your past bad options and understand what you can do in a different manner, which takes humility.

Wisdom also gives you the chance to identify the difference between reversible and irreversible decisions. Then, you can permit yourself to make well-informed and bold risks. You can also make mistakes without any fear or hesitations. Whenever you commit simple or complex blunders, you can take them as constructive criticism for your professional and personal development.

Fear of failure has been associated with conservative and slow decision. Poor life choices can even affect the quality of your thoughts. Instead of feeling afraid to commit mistakes, you should have at least tried. What if something great happened? When the result is not what you expected in the first place, it's still a perfect way to grow as a professional.

Let's say you have a new and fresh idea for an upcoming event in the company or organization you're currently working. Imagine your colleagues or superiors reject your idea. So, what will happen next? While some would feel hopeless, it's better to improve on your thought, make a research, and offer it to other businesses.

If the result is the same, reflect again. Do you think you overlook something important? Study and develop your ideas. Even you fail a thousand times, keep your sight in reaching all your dreams. Although you are lost in the midst of your journey, visualize your objectives.

Keep your Overconfidence in Check

Do you know that overconfidence can make your judgment and reasoning awry? Recent studies and research indicate that people are likely to overestimate the accuracy of their knowledge and their performance.

Perhaps, you are 90% certain you can convince your superiors to promote you. Or maybe, you are 100% sure you know your ideas can lead to huge business success. If you're overconfident about such things, your plans will go awry.

It's imperative to consider the level of your confidence when it comes to time management. Many of us tend to overestimate how much we can achieve within a short period of time. Do you think finishing your report will only take an hour or two? Do you believe that you can pay your bills within a few minutes? You might be overconfident in all your predictions.

Before anything else, spend time to estimate the chance of your success rate. Then, review and examine your estimates. Ask if your thought is as accurate as you imagined. Remember that good decision maker and critical thinkers recognize in their lives that overconfidence could be a big predicament. Then, adjust your behavior and way of thinking.

Identify Every Risk You Take

Familiarity always leads to comfort, and it's risky to make poor decisions. It's because you probably are accustomed to your weak habits. You even don't think about all the dangers along the way.

For example, you might drive at a high speed to come to your destination before your shift starts. Let's say you always arrive in the office without a traffic or ticket violation. As time passes by, you get more comfortable with fast driving. However, the truth is that you jeopardize your safety, and you take a legal risk.

Another good example is when you eat fast food every day. Since you don't see signs of serious complications, you might not consider it a big problem. But you may experience health issues or gain weight in the long run.

The secret here is to determine the habits that you become accustomed to. Why? It's because these are the things that require your attention. After that, assess whether your decisions are unhealthy or harmful. Then, create and develop a plan to have good habits.

Chapter 8: How to See More Clearly?

Clear thinking is not something that many people instinctually do. It cannot be denied that humans look for pleasure, food, survival, and sex. Everything else that a person views as a higher pursuit is only second. This is where mental models can come into play, ensuring that we think clearly and critically. Bear in mind that the world looks different at a second or third glance.

Clear thinking sounds simple to achieve. But the truth is that it is easier said than done and mental models make everything less stressful and more challenging. In the previous chapters, we have learned that mental models can help an individual make better decision making. Clear thinking is no exception.

To perceive the world as accurately as possible and think at your best, there are various things to do or consider. At first, it's confusing where to start, and neophytes have a higher risk to fail. But it doesn't necessarily mean that experienced individuals can handle the process effectively. People of all ages would have a hard time to think clearly and critically. In this chapter, we will learn how to see more clearly to help us face our daily challenges well and avoid stressful consequences over time. Are you ready? Let's get started!

Ignore Black Swan

The first thing to think clearly is to ignore black swans. You probably have heard of black swans before. But what does it mean? How does it work? And what makes ignoring black swans beneficial?

A black swan is simple and unpredictable event, which has severe consequences and is beyond what you expect in the first place. A black swan event is characterized by its rarity, impact, and the practice of explaining a failure.

A black swan is considered a rare event with serious results. Although many people claim it to be predictable, others say that it cannot be predicted in advance. Any black swan events can even result in catastrophic effect to a specific economy. Since they are not predictable, it's possible to be prepared by building strong and effective systems. Of course, most of us will rely on forecasting tools. But the truth is that the use of such solutions can fail to predict and boost vulnerability to black swans. More particularly, it can increase risk and provide inefficient security.

Black Swan was popularized or coined by Nassim Nicholas Taleb who is a finance professor, former Wall Street trader, and writer. Prior to the 2008 financial crisis, Taleb wrote the black swan event in 2007. *"Since a black swan event is impossible to foresee because of its catastrophic consequences and extreme rarity, people need to assume that it's always possible. Then, extensive research and a careful planning can play a critical role,"* he argued.

For rare events, the tools of prediction and probability don't apply because they depend on the past sample sizes and large population. Extrapolating based on observations of past events is not useful as well. It can even pose a potential risk to us.

Nowadays, the experienced team ignores the early signs of black swans. Then, they move forward into their goals despite the problems. Why do you think individuals ignore a black swan event? It's because it can help clear their minds, materialize an event, and prepare them for a chaotic problem in the coming years.

Look for Equilibrium Point

Another mental model to see more clearly is to look for an equilibrium point. For the past years, the number of ways to visualize the concept has been skyrocketing. But the one that comes from Boombustology is the simplest and the most effective solution to use. How does it work? Or what makes it different from others? Well, it's where a ball sits on a curved shape.

Equilibrium is possible when the ball itself find its unique location. This is especially true when it's left to its devices. Overshooting and undershooting the location can be self-correcting. Disequilibrium, on the contrary, happens when the ball cannot find its location. That's not all! The ball cannot generate a self-correcting move. Disequilibrium can generate self-reinforcing motion, which accelerates the ball's move away from such a stable state.

Equilibrium is also considered a balance between opposing forces. Just like the variety of mental models, there are various types of equilibrium as well. You probably have heard about static equilibrium. Perhaps, you also encountered dynamic equilibrium. What's the difference between the two terms?

When a system is at rest, it's called a static equilibrium. When two or more forces are well-matched, it means dynamic equilibrium.

A scale, for example, with equal weight on both sides, show static equilibrium. Let's say you fill a bathtub with water. Then, you turn the faucet off, which shows static equilibrium.

However, the time you unplug the drain or turn on the faucet, it's simply a dynamic equilibrium.

Another example of equilibrium is the rule of supply and demand. Warren Buffet, the founder of Berkshire Hathaway, bought approximately 11.2 million ounces of silver.

"For the past years, bullion inventories have declined. Last summer, Charlie and I came up with a conclusion that a higher price can play a big role in establishing the equilibrium between the supply and demand," Buffet said.

The only way to restore the market with a good state of equilibrium was to raise the prices. Known as the balancing force to supply, demand can also result in a successful and lasting investment. With the knowledge of supply and demand, you can make a better investment decision. You perhaps are thinking of the producers of an aluminum can and other undifferentiated goods. However, they are a poor investment simply because they can only lead to sufficient returns when the supply is tight. When there's excess capacity in the sector, the price rate will decline, and only the owners are left with poor returns on investment.

The low cost producers are the only winners. As prices decrease, they are the ones who can maintain production. Then, high-cost competitors should cut the production to reduce the supply and moves the sector to equilibrium. When everything is back to normal, the production is no exception. However, the low cost producers are single people who can operate throughout the cycle.

Profit opportunities from equilibrium only take place when the demand exceeds the capacity, which in turn can lead to a positive or negative change in demand and supply. Although this equilibrium is simple, it remains incomplete, but we should consider reflexivity.

"Reflexivity helps shape all participants' thinking, which can develop the reality throughout the process. Although both thinking and reality approach each other, they would never be identical at the end of the day," George Soros writes.

Think with System 2

Daniel Kahneman's best-selling book entitled Thinking, Fast and Slow tackles about the two modes of thought such as the System 1 and System 2. What is the difference between the two terms?

The system 1 is fast, frequent, stereotypic, emotional, and unconscious. It can identify that a specific object is at a greater distance compared to other things, find the source of a sound, read different texts on a billboard, make a good chess move, and understand sentences.

Below are the other things they can perform:

- Display disgust every time they see a terrible image.
- Solve basic addition.
- Drive a vehicle, especially on an empty road.

System 2, on the contrary, is slow, logical, conscious, calculating, infrequent, and effortful. It can direct your interest especially to the clowns and other performers at the circus. It can help dig in your memory to recognize every sound, identify an appropriate behavior during a formal gathering, park into a tight space, identify the validity of a logical reasoning, and more.

Here are the other things that the system 2 can do:

- Brace yourself before the beginning of a sprint.
- Direct your attention to a person at a party.
- Look out for an individual with grey hair.
- Sustain an above-average walking rate.
- Ascertain both the quality and price of an appliance.
- Solve more complex multiplication equation.

So, which is better between System 1 and System 2 for you to see more clearly? Well, think with the latter to make a logical decision making. No matter how difficult a situation you face along the way, System 2 can make you reasonable at all times.

After decades of extensive research and contribution to a range of fields, Daniel Kahneman won the Nobel Memorial Prize in Economic Sciences. He also received the National Academies Communication Award for his work, which helps the public to understand engineering, medicine, behavioral science, and other fields.

As with looking for equilibrium point and ignoring a black swan event, thinking with system 2 takes a long time and practice. Although this mode of thought is slower, it is driven by logic and deliberation. Furthermore, System 2 can drive many of your life choices.

Chapter 9: Learning Organization

As a term, a learning organization is given to a company or business that facilitates the learning of their employees so that the former would continue to grow in the industry. Learning organization exists due to the pressure that small- or big-sized companies face for the past years to remain competitive and productive in the sector. Coined by Peter Senge and his colleagues, learning organization leads to an interconnected and effective way of thinking. Such companies become a community, in which all employees feel committed to help the former realize their goals. Over the years, the concept is hailed as a panacea for a business success in a diverse and complicated economy. Due to the complexity or uncertainty of the environment, the concept remains increasingly relevant to all parts of the industry. *"The rate at which businesses of all sizes learn may serve as a sustainable and effective source of advantage,"* Senge said.

While the idea seems inspiring, people find it hard to implement and incorporate. It involves a profound change in the employees' mind. The organization's culture and society are no exception. Also, such a change is a long and stressful process. It does not happen in a snap. Aside from ample time, it requires your attention, effort, and other resources.

What is a learning organization in a deeper sense?

- *"Learning organizations are organizations where all professionals expand their capacity to turn their expected results into a reality. It's where new patterns of thinking are fostered, and aspiration is set free,"* Peter Senge added.

- *"Learning organization is an organization with the philosophy for anticipating and responding to both complexity and uncertainty."*

- According to McGill, together with his colleagues, a learning organization is a company that can effectively respond to information by changing their programming.

- A learning organization is a company that can modify its perspectives and behaviors due to their years of experience and wide expertise. While this sounds an obvious statement, most organizations are unable to acknowledge the facts and repeat the same behavior.

These days, the competition is tough while the market is changing and uncertain. That's why any organizations need to survive and grow. Obviously, managers have a lot of responsibilities to perform. Using their skill and sound judgment, they have to make the right decisions when a problem takes place. Effective decision making requires businesses of all sizes to develop and enhance their ability of learning behaviors within a short span of time. This new insight into a startup or big companies is considered a fighting process when facing the pace of change. Throughout this procedure, managers should increase both the awareness and the employee's ability to understand or manage both the environment and the organization itself. In this case, they can make smart decisions, secure the company, and make their objectives happen. Nowadays, managers guarantee organizational learning. However, they are unable to understand how to make and develop their company a learning organization.

Both groups and individuals learn. This is especially true when there are well-designed systems and conditions. They can share new learning across the company and incorporate it into its existing practices and culture.

People who have a leadership role in a learning organization act as a designer, steward, and teacher to establish a shared vision and challenge existing mental models. They are responsible for learning while the employees are expanding all their capabilities to become more competitive in the coming years.

The basic concept for a learning organization is that only flexible and adaptive companies will excel during emergency situations. In this case, the businesses themselves need to improve employees' dedication and ability to learn at different levels.

With a goal to bring new ideas, the learning organization also aims to debate current issues, introduce effective strategies, and provide timely case studies.

At present, professionals in different fields consider learning organization a process. Over time, the concept of a learning organization as an apolitical end-state will gain acceptance in different parts of the globe.

What's the key factor in building a successful learning organization? Well, it relies on how the companies process their managerial expertise and experience. The ability of a startup or big businesses is not measured by what they know. It's assessed by how they learn instead. Management practices also encourage creativity, empathy, systematic thinking, and a sense of efficacy.

Although every employee can learn, the working environment is not conducive to proactive engagement and holistic reflection. That's not all! Everyone lacks the tools and other guiding ideas to handle daily situations and challenges. Aside from ensuring success in a business operation, the learning organization aims to create and develop a good future for employees and other concerned individuals.

The mastery of basic disciplines makes a learning organization different from the conventional organization. Peter Senge's five disciplines are converging to transform a learning organization into a more innovative company, according to experts. These can include Building a Shared vision, systems thinking, mental models, team learning, and personal mastery.

A Simple Overview of Senge's Five Disciplines

"Approximately one-third of 500 businesses will disappear in 15 years. The lifetime for the largest companies, on the contrary, is around 40 decades," Peter Senge said. This concept enables today's organizations to experience constant growth, perform effectively, and stand out from the competition.

Rather than visualizing a conventional hierarchy, companies can address the challenges when they create a strong and effective learning organization. Senge's five disciplines describe the proper way of managing a business' success or development. They also give everyone an idea of how employees exceed their company's expectations.

5 Disciplines of Senge's Learning Organizations

1. Building a Shared Vision

In every learning organization, those with leadership goals should create and develop the vision together with the employees. Most leaders have personal objectives. However, they don't share it to the lifeblood of any business – employees.

By compromising the company's and employee's goals, it's possible to create a shared vision. With that, turning a business performance into a learning mechanism and changing the relationship will be a reality.

2. Systems Thinking

The learning organizations was developed from systems thinking, a conceptual framework, which enables everyone to study businesses. Whether you evaluate a company or has ample information systems, learning organization uses this system thinking. This Sense's discipline states that every character should be visible in a company, making it a learning organization. But what will happen when these characters are missing? Simply, business falls short of its objectives.

But some experts believe that the characteristics are gradually acquired. In simple terms, they are not developed simultaneously.

Servers as the cornerstone of a learning organization, system thinking integrate employees of a business, making them a body of theory or practice.

Rather than focusing on specific issues, this discipline indicates the process of a whole system. That's why anyone with leadership rules should remember that both action and outcomes are correlated with one another.

Sometimes, managers only focus on specific actions, which in turn can result in overlooking the big picture. But when they understand the correlation, system thinking allows us to see the relationship of change in a specific situation. They will also identify the cause and effect of every problem along the way.

3. Mental Models

Called as ingrained assumptions or generalizations, mental models influence how we take action and understand the things that surround us.

To make the shift to a learning organization fast, it's important to challenge these mental models. In this fast-paced world, individuals are likely to adopt theories. In most cases, businesses have memories that preserve behaviors, values, and norms.

When establishing a learning environment, adopt an open culture to promote trust, and replace any confrontational attitudes. To realize this goal, the mechanisms for identifying and evaluating organizational theories are highly imperative.

The mental models begin when they turn the mirror inward. Simply, we are capable of unearthing internal pictures about the world, which hold them to scrutiny. More than that, it includes the skill to continue any meaningful conversations, balancing advocacy, and inquiry.

If businesses of all sizes develop the ability to work with this discipline, the workforce needs to acquire sets of skills and improve new orientations. But institutional changes and openness in a company can be critical.

4. Team Learning

Individual learning encompasses of team learning, which allows the employees to grow professionally. With access to expertise and knowledge, it can improve the organization's problem solving capacity. A learning organization is packed with structures that encourage team learning with openness, boundary-crossing, and other features. Team learning also requires individuals of different levels to engage in discussion. However, team members need to foster open communication, shared insights, and shared meaning as well. A learning organization has superb knowledge management structures, which can lead to the creation, acquisition, and implementation of the knowledge in the business of all sizes.

A lot of organizations also view team learning as the process of aligning or developing a specific team's capacities to achieve their expected results. Not only can it build on personal mastery, but it can also lead to a shared vision. Unfortunately, these are not enough. All employees should work together to maximize good outcomes and guarantee personal development in the long run.

The concept of team learning begins with a dialogue and the member's capacity to stop assumptions and make genuine thinking.

The idea of team learning among a company's employees supports them to be open-minded to the flow of wider and greater intelligence. Combined with systems thinking, every dialogue can create a suitable and relevant language to deal with any complexity. Instead of being diverted by questions of leadership style, everyone can focus on structural forces and other issues.

5. **Personal Mastery**

When a person clearly visualizes his goals with a perception of reality, personal mastery takes place. What drives the employees to practice all activities to make their objectives happen? The gap between reality and vision encourages them to go beyond their limitations.

However, this tension depends on how a professional understands an existing reality. Sharing the truth is an important fundamental for this Senge's discipline. But a business' employees could believe they lack the skills to realize their objectives. *"We should spend time to train and bring the potential of our subconscious mind to handle complex problems as effectively as possible,"* Peter Senge said.

Why is a Learning Organization of High Importance?

Rather than relying on ad hoc process to achieve organizational learning thru serendipity, a learning organization encourages and boosts collective learning. While it can maximize successful business results, it can provide other advantages and here are some of them:

- Small- or medium-sized companies can remain competitive and productive in the industry despite the competition. They can also keep a high level of innovation and incorporate new trends into their business.

- They can respond to new and external pressures. They can become flexible and effective, enabling them to provide the best services to various and potential clients.

- A learning organization can enable businesses to link their existing resources to their customers' growing and changing needs.

- It improves the quality of outputs and services at different levels. Despite the difficulty of every stage, products or services will remain responsive and relevant.

- It improves the image of a company and makes it people-oriented over time. From building brand awareness to establishing a good reputation, the possibilities are endless.

- It also increases the pace of change in startups and other businesses. The industry is changing. But it's hard to incorporate that change into a business. With a learning organization, it lessens the complexities, makes the process simple, and guarantee success.

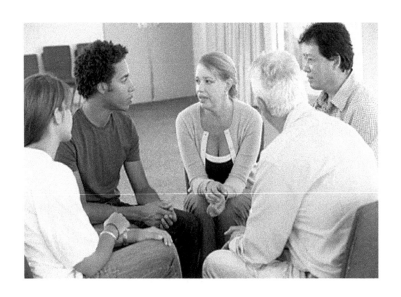

Chapter 10: Become One with Nature

Classic science is more likely to consider nature as something external to regulate and foresee. Scientists try to know the forces of nature and harness them for the gain of humanity. That usage of nature could be positive, which result in different technological innovations that save lives and make living simpler.

The initial phase in joining our body, along with nature, is thinking that we are part of nature. We are not separate from it, but we are a vital part of it all. Our body is composed of all the same energy, elements, and minerals, which creates our planet. The majority of scholars and quantum physicists think that all things in the outer universe are only a mirror of our consciousness as well as our body. For instance, the ratio of water in the Earth mirrors the similar ratio of water within our bodies and more.

It is a fact that people are nature-beings. However, we could still fall out of arrangement along with our natural characters. You see, wellness is in melody with nature. It supports ourselves with the innate understanding, which is within everybody.

For instance, we get tired for a specific time at night that is the natural circadian rhythm of the body that works. No matter if you like to go to sleep at a particular time, it is always up to you. Most of the time, not listening to the cues of your body could be the difference between sickness and health.

One research tells that what everybody feels and knows lessens stress. It's also believed that spending some time in nature is considered anti-inflammatory. The experts discovered that positive emotions felt with nature are connected to low levels of pro-inflammatory cytokines.

If we connect with ourselves, the outdoors, and the signals of our body are the answer in optimal well-being.

Below are some ways so you can connect your body along with nature.

Become one with the elements

It could be swimming in the sea or simply camping in the forest. These simple ways could get you into nature. You must understand about the different minerals and crystals as well as their healing abilities. You could also learn the various animals, flowers and plants and every creature of life.

Feel the air and breathe it in a place abundant with trees. You can also climb a mountain or a boulder. Silently listen to the birds. The sweet sounds of nature and the wind in the trees. Perform meditative types of movement like yoga, qi gong, and tai chi in nature.

Start imagining the roots mounting into the earth from your arms and your feet as the twigs of the tree. You can think of what fruits you bare and what it's grounded into. Visualize you're an eagle in the blue sky. Where would you like to go, and how would you feel? Picture yourself if you are one of your favorite animals. Can you feel their vitality inside your form?

1. **Listen to what your body tells**

   Listening to your body is very simple. When you are feeling tired, sleep. If you are starving and craving for food, eat. If you are feeling invigorated, move your body. If you are suffering from pain, listen up, and ask why. You might not know, but it might be that you need some massage. Perhaps you need to stretch more and slowdown from everything you do.

2. **Exercise moon and sun gazing**

   Everyone loves to look up at the moon at night. However, have you ever tried to look for a long time and feel the connection with the brightest thing in the night sky? You understand that the moon is accountable for variations in the seas low and high tides. Are you aware that the moon has a massive impact on your emotional condition too? In fact, a woman's menstrual cycle is directly influenced by the waning and waxing of the moon.

   On the other hand, sun gazing is a fascinating exercise, which has been practiced for many centuries. Several individuals even report not wanting any food by just staring into the sun during particular times of the day.

You see, throughout those times, the sun doesn't have any negative impacts on the eyes. It's also believed in boosting eyesight, vitality, and energy as well.

3. **Feel the ground**

In case you didn't know yet, your skin breathes and absorbs minerals and vitamins from the planet. For instance, when you go barefoot on the ocean, the negative ions from the salts in the sea and sand are known to have healing powers on one's body. What's more, try digging your feet into the soil, as it's also known to have benefits. You must allow your feet's skin to touch the ground, the grass, and the sea.

4. **Gazing the clouds and the stars**

Staring upward could be a means to exceed space-time truth. The majority of civilizations stared to the stars to seek power and guidance. Are you familiar with the expression, *"as above, so below?"*

Everyone is composed of stardust. Understanding about the stars could bring us above the mundane and into optimum consciousness. Meanwhile, cloud gazing is, no doubt a fun type of meditation. Stare at the sky above so you can have that pure energy.

5. **Transform your mindset**

You must understand that nature is not simple on the outside in your environment. You are part of that being too! The identical water, which pours in the sea, also runs over your bloodstream. The similar minerals and seas you see in nature are the substance from which your body and bones are developed. What's more, the air you breathe is a type of symbiotic connection between trees and humans. That offers the crucial element for one another to flourish and live.

Always remember that your body is built from nature. You present your physical body back to nature at the end of the incarnation. When you perform meditation, and you continuously go outdoors physically, you connect along with your extended body.

As you can see, you can now tap into any part of nature, as it's innately within you. No matter how long you like to stay inside your room, under the fluorescent light or at your desk, you cannot deny the fact that you are nature. Nothing could take that away from you.

Lightning Source UK Ltd.
Milton Keynes UK
UKHW020657040621
384928UK00011B/779